The Death Sentence Of Valley Fever (Coccidioidomycosis)

Quality Of Life Through Observations From Author And Valley Fever Survivor D. Waters

Copyright © 2019 by D. Waters

All rights reserved. This book or any portion thereof may not be reproduced or used in any matter whatsoever without the express written permission of the author except for a brief quotation for use in a book review.

First printing 2019

ISBN: 9781092891905

Editing and cover design provided by

Young Waters Studio

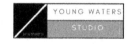

Whisper House Publishing

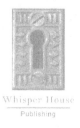

www.WhisperHousePublishing.com

For Angie,
The best part of my day.

And Joe the dog—
My purpose.

- CHAPTER 1 1
  - TEAS 13
  - NEEM LEAF & OLIVE LEAF TEA 13
  - PAU D'ARCO BARK & BARBERRY LEAF TEA 14
  - GINGER ROOT TEA 14
  - FINAL TEA COMBINATION 15
- CHAPTER 2 16
  - COCONUT CURRY LENTIL SOUP 20
  - ROASTED BRUSSEL SPROUTS 21
  - ROASTED CAULIFLOWER STEAKS 22
  - ASPARAGAS 23
  - SPICY AYOLI SAUCE 24
- CHAPTER 3 25
  - SPINACH – BACON – EGG SALAD 27
  - WATERMELON JUICE 33
  - TUNA SALAD 35
- CHAPTER 4 36
  - CAULIFLOWER PIZZA CRUST 40
  - GARLIC PARMESAN SPAGHETTI SQUASH 42
- CHAPTER 5 44
  - LENTILS – BASIC 47
  - BEEF STRIPS 49
- CONCLUSION 50
- APPENDIX I

Chapter 1

Athletic, active and surpassing many physical goals and accomplishments. Running farther, faster than I could've ever imagined, this was my life as a young boy.

As a teen, I surfed the local beaches of my hometown in Southern California. My mother cooked healthy meals (she was somewhat health-conscious before health-conscious was trendy). This fueled my active life. Surfing daily, always on the go, I never tired.

In my twenties good health was a constant even though my life's path brought me to heroin addiction, crime and lengthy prison sentences in the California and Federal prison system. You can read more details of my adventurous life in my critically acclaimed autobiography, I Slept Through the American Dream by D. Waters. Available on Amazon.

Learn more at www.WhisperHousePublishing.com.

With all my self-inflicted struggles and hurdles now behind me and after conquering near-death experiences and bucking the odds of survival, I was now fifty-two years old. Life became unbelievably good, to the point of surreal at times, with a feeling of peacefulness which allowed me to enjoy my life to the fullest. Still active, physical and competitive, I felt like a young man again, being free from life's major obstacles. I now had solutions for challenging hurdles that everyday life gives us, or as I say, "Life throws us curveballs; you just have to learn to hit a curve."

Over the next decade plus years, I was doing the desires of my heart, camping on the coast of California and hiking the inland hills overlooking the Pacific Ocean. Although I was sixty-five, I felt like I still had an edge over most, not only people of my age but also many years younger. I attribute this to my constant physical movement and my conscious awareness of my good eating habits. I was getting a second chance in life and I could see myself riding off into the sunset. Compared to my previous lifestyle of bad decisions, the thought process of expecting the unexpected was erased from my mind.

Then almost overnight I didn't feel good, in fact I started feeling terrible. Yes, I was older (65) and I understand the slowing down coming with age, but I knew this was something more than that. Basically, I've never been to the doctor, never suffered broken bones and have always believed that we know our bodies better than anyone, so I had no reason to ever seek medical help. But now, I knew something was wrong!

Not feeling good happened more abruptly than at a gradual pace over time. I would notice in the mornings my legs would be extremely stiff, as well as my leg muscles would be in a semi-cramped stage until I moved around for a short period of time. I contributed this all to my age, but the suddenness of pain did concern me. Along with a runny nose and a lack of motivation throughout the day, I passed it off as a flu bug or some small virus that was zapping my energy, feeling confident it would pass within a couple of days. Time went by and I wasn't getting any better. Along with headaches and my breathing being compromised, I just kept pushing through each and every day. At this point the thought of a basic check up by a doctor never crossed my mind. I started sitting in the house more and more having to prepare myself mentally to do my daily tasks. I can remember many times having to get pumped up mentally just to go empty the trash. My once active physical self wasn't inspired to do any of the things that I enjoyed doing so much in the past. This went on for months and my condition worsened with the pain a lot more prominent, extreme fatigue and I was developing small, blotchy red rash spots on my legs as well as my lower torso. Finally, I made an appointment to go see a general practitioner. My appointment to see the doctor was approximately a month away now, and within that month I felt daily drained.

Negativity breeds negativity, and I stopped looking forward to anything throughout the day. As I awoke in the morning I would force myself to push through it all, but I was losing the battle. A good day would consist of a shower and being able to get most of my simple daily chores done. But many days all I could do was wake up, sit for a couple of hours and lie back down. My attitude had become questionable because of the pain and not knowing what was going on. Mentally I was playing ping-pong in my brain with thoughts of my life coming to an end, or worse, living a lengthy life in the state I was in now. The negativity was breeding at a rapid pace.

At my initial doctor visit I had a laundry list of questions; I just wanted to know what was causing me to feel this way. After checking my vitals, and a few questions of his own, he scheduled me for blood tests as well as x-rays. I realize the medical process of narrowing down the medical problem, but I also wanted something concrete to wrap my head around as being the cause of my change in health. Optimism has always been a strong suit of mine, as well as being a positive person from having common sense and logic, but I couldn't make heads or tails of what was going on.

I wanted a starting point so I could deal with the situation. During the time of waiting for my blood work and x-rays to come back I still was not feeling any better, maybe even worse. Back in the doctor's office with my test results, he said he wanted more lab work and also a tuberculosis test. I was really pushing the doctor to give me something more tangible because it was coming up on six months since I started feeling different, and my condition was taking any form of enjoyment from my life. He (the doctor) did mention on my x-rays my lungs were very spotty, so naturally I asked him what did he think that was caused from; although he hesitated he said he felt strongly that it was probably lung cancer. Lung cancer, I thought to myself this is not good. My girlfriend always accompanies me to my doctor visits and when she heard this news she had tears in her eyes. Although I felt like I was kicked by a mule from his medically educated diagnosis, I also realized that I smoked cigarettes for much of my adult life, so lung cancer made complete sense even though it was not what I wanted to hear. The doctor wanted to rule out tuberculosis completely so he gave me a second TB test. I left the office that day dumbfounded, but at the same time it was something definite that I could put my finger on. I pride myself on being a good listener but that day with the confusion of a life-threatening disease in the form of cancer rolling around in my head I didn't hear the word probably like I should have if I would have been paying attention.

Now, every day there was a mood of sadness around my house from the devastating news of a terminal illness. It was not death that bothered me, it was the idea that I would become dependent on others and bring their life down in the process. I know that medical research had made a lot of progress with cancer remedies which generated some hope.

Back again at the doctor's office to find out the results of the second series of tests, I wanted to start whatever I needed to do in hopes of getting better. To my surprise the doctor wanted more tests, a third tuberculosis test which was different from the first two, which were a small needle prick under my skin in the forearm area. He ordered blood test pertaining to tuberculosis so he could eliminate this disease completely. He also had me see a specialist, a pulmonologist for oxygen capacity in my lungs, as well as another series of x-rays. During all this testing and waiting I had made no improvements in how I felt.

I wasn't telling anyone of my lung cancer diagnosis except for a couple of close friends. I've never been a man searching for pity, and really didn't need to be asked how I was feeling on a daily basis by casual acquaintances or even strangers. For me, this just reminds me that I'm sick to the point of giving power to the illness. I knew I was sick, but I also knew the character of person that I had become in life, which made me determined to make the best out of bad situations, all bad situations! Before leaving the doctor's office that day he did state that he positively thought it was 99% that I had lung cancer.

Now returning to the pulmonologist's office I disclosed to him that my primary physician had diagnosed me with lung cancer. He said he wasn't completely in agreement with that diagnosis. The runny nose and rash on parts of my body didn't fit with the lung cancer prognosis. And the pulmonologist ordered yet another blood test, as well as a CAT scan. Which he said would give him more information to identify what was actually causing my lungs to look spotty. Frustrated in the fact that no one was getting to the solution of my daily pain, and limited activity, I completed this new series of tests and started the waiting process for the results. My general health was reaching an all-time low, and daily I struggled mentally as well as physically to get through another day, while trying not to bring down the other people in my life with my physical burden. These were very bad days for sure.

The pulmonologist's office called me telling me they needed to see me as soon as possible. I went back with the idea of more of the same, wanting more blood, no precise answers and probably expecting to have to do a series of more tests. But what the doctor (pulmonologist) told me was completely different than I had imagined. He stated that I have Coccidioidomycosis, or cocci, commonly known as Valley Fever. Now I was really thrown for a loop since I had no idea what any of these words meant. He further went on to explain that Coccidioidomycosis is caused by tiny spores from a fungus called coccidioides-immitis. The spores are carried from the soil into the air by the wind or disturbances in the dirt ranging from construction to earthquakes. In many instances, symptoms never materialize and people don't get sick. Other cases can cause flu-like signs and sometimes a red, spotty rash. The symptoms can develop into chronic pneumonia or other long-term issues.

I only had one question that day, "Are you 100% sure of what you are telling me?"

He stated, "100% since your tests confirming Valley Fever were sent to a specialized lab before I knew the results to be positive for cocci."

He continued, treatment involves antifungal medication taken for several months or longer, depending on the severity of the symptoms. In rare and potentially fatal incidents, the illness can spread from the lungs to the brain and spinal cord, spawning complications like meningitis.

The contaminated area which has the fungus causing Coccidioidomycosis is only in the Southwest region of the United States. This he told me Mr. Waters is what you contracted and that is why you feel the way you feel, as well as explaining the rash and spots on my lungs along with the pain.

The pulmonologist went on to say he had received a copy of the letter from the local public health department registering me with the state because I had a reportable fungal disease, a formality the county does after receiving blood test results positive for Coccidioidomycosis. Valley Fever is reportable in over half the states in the U.S.. State health departments collect information about cases of Valley Fever and then send the information to CDC through the National Notifiable Diseases Surveillance System (NNDSS).

At home that day, after leaving the pulmonologist's office, I didn't know what to think. In some ways the lung cancer seemed like a better chance of survival, thinking that at least they had made some progress in treating cancer. This mysterious disease of Valley Fever that I was diagnosed with to me seemed like a conundrum to the doctors as well as to science. Incurable, relatively rare as well as the vague treatment of this disease left me not knowing which way to turn.

Going back to my original doctor, my general practitioner, I let him know of my Coccidioidomycosis. Oddly enough the next thing he asked was what prisons had I been in? I said many, do you want them in chronological order or alphabetical order. So the first penitentiary I mentioned was a state prison in northern California, Vacaville. He matter-of-factly said, "That's probably where you got it!"

I replied, "How could you possibly know that?" And I added,"That was many years ago, I've been to many other prisons and places since then."

He just kept saying how he felt strongly that was the location in which I contracted Valley Fever. I've learned since that prisons have a high rate of cocci within the South West region. Thirteen Californian prisoners had died in 2016 alone.

Then I let the doctor know that I wasn't concerned at all where I got infected, but what we can do about it now so I can feel better, and get on the right side of this thing. He reiterated what the pulmonologist had told me, no cure because of not being able to kill the fungus growing inside you. My thoughts were bleak but I was determined to do something, even if it was wrong, to just do something to fight. The doctor told me one of my options was with medication, 200 mg of fluconazole twice a day could maybe slow down the growth of fungus., that through my x-rays and CAT scan, showed prominent on my lungs as well as my spleen and liver.

Trusting the doctor because of his medical education, yet skeptical from his lack of knowledge of this disease, I left his office that day with a prescription of fluconazole, as well as vitamin D, fifty thousand units to be taken twice a week, along with an appointment to be seen by him again in three months.

I consider myself to be a very fortunate man these days for so many reasons, and one of the main reasons is I have a girlfriend, Angie, who deeply cares about my well-being. She also understands that I don't do things without investigating the pluses and minuses of major decisions. Also, I am blessed in the fact that Angie's department of expertise is research. For years she has done information gathering for major corporations, and I might add very successfully. In addition, I know that sometimes side effects from medication can outweigh the benefits and can cause one to feel worse. So, when I was given a prescription for fluconazole, Angie and I researched its known side effects. What I found out is that fluconazole can cause stomach problems, headaches, dizziness along with hair loss, extreme tiredness, nausea and even negatively affect the liver.

So my personal choice was to take the medication, (fluconazole) and pay attention to how my body reacted to any or all of the side effects. I was physically feeling so bad that I was almost willing to try anything. At this point every day was worse than the day before physically, so I felt highly confident that if the medication is going to impact me positively I would feel the effects and realize that it was working. But what I didn't realize and I realize it now, the medication wasn't to make me feel better but rather to slow down or stop the growth of the fungus on my internal organs. And with time I might not keep feeling worse with a slight chance of feeling only a little better.

After a couple of months of the fluconazole treatment, I basically felt about the same, and some days I felt the medication was not helping, but adding to the problem with some of the side effects. I was so tired on a daily basis along with excruciating headaches that I couldn't separate the Valley Fever from the fluconazole. One day my friend Stevie D. was picking me up to go get some coffee, when climbing up into his truck he noticed my awkwardness and strain caused from being in wrenching pain.

Steve was aware of my Coccidioidomycosis and simply asked me, "Do you think you will always feel like this?"

"Yes I think I will," was my reply.

I didn't think much of that conversation until a couple of days later. Then the clarity of the situation hit me. I reflected on my past challenging lifestyle and how I had overcome the curveballs thrown at me with the help from others as well as my positive drive and competitive spirit. With my life experiences, I knew I had the ability to change; to not live in the problem, and to live in the solution. This is what I needed to do now. Although I didn't know how I would do it, I did know for a fact, that I could do it.

Realizing that I didn't physically feel like taking walks, hiking or any form of exercise, I needed to attack the disease in its origin, internally. So through research, Angie and I started to form some plan of attack and bring the battle to the fungus inside of me. I felt if I could arrest the fungus it would give me that boost I needed to take on more physical activity. To me, this would be giving a one-two punch to the Coccidioidomycosis that was robbing me of life.

Common sense told me water in quantity would be a good starting point. I started to drink 1 L bottles of water two to three times a day. I prefer Smart brand water or an alkaline based water, but it's your preference. I would add one pack of Emergen-C in at least one of the 1 L waters I would drink throughout the day. Emergen-C packs contain 1000 mg of vitamin C, and can be found in most supermarkets or drugstores. Also I found aloe vera juice through my research could also help. I would add approximately 1/3 of a 16.9 fluid ounce bottle of aloe vera juice to my 1 L drinks. I found a product called Aleo Vita which comes in many flavors and also available at most supermarkets. When drinking large amounts of water the body can lose much-needed electrolytes, so the Emergen-C packs can help replace your body's electrolyte loss. Once in a while I will have a Gatorade to replenish my body's electrolytes, but because of the sugar this was rare. Note: aloe vera juice is excellent for critical body detox and best drank on an empty stomach. So in the morning the first thing I have is this mixture of water, vitamin C and aloe vera to get my system started, approximately 8 to 10 ounces.

Then I went to a body detoxification form of tea. The ingredients are Bareberry Root C/S, Neem Leaf C/S, Pau D'Arco Bark C/S, and Olive Leaf Cut. I add fresh grated ginger to balance out the bitterness of the tea. The brand of tea I use is Starwest Botanicals, but once again, it's your preference on brand.

I wanted to avoid going into too much scientific detail, so I also need to advise you to use your common sense when using medicinal herbs. One issue when using herbs is the difficulty to find dosage information, so I advise that any medicinal herb should be ingested with caution. Keep in mind that natural products are not always necessarily safe and dosages can be important. Be sure to follow relevant directions on product labels and consult your pharmacist or physician or other healthcare professional before using. More detailed information and warnings on the herbs are in Appendix.

Below are some ingredient highlights of the detox tea. In choosing these herbs, I looked for treatments that had an indication for treating fungal disorders, reducing inflammation, and promoting immune health. This is by no means comprehensive, but offered as a starting point for you.

NEEM LEAF

Benefits of neem leaves include immunomodulatory, anti-inflammatory, antihyperglycaemic, antiulcer, antimalarial, antifungal, antibacterial, antiviral, antioxidant, antimutagenic and anticarcinogenic properties.

OLIVE LEAVES

Research shows oleuropein, the main component in olive leaf extract, has antioxidant, antibacterial, antimicrobial, anti-inflammatory, and immune-stimulating properties.

PAU D' ARCO BARK

In herbal medicine, extracts of the pau d'arco bark have long been used to treat a wide range of medical disorders. The information I found pointed to it helping reduce inflammation and infection. What interested me is that the bark is highly resistant to rotting, mold, and other common tree pathogens. It has long been presumed that these antimicrobial properties may be beneficial to humans, either by preventing or treating common bacterial, viral, or fungal infections.

BARBERRY ROOT

The Chinese have used berberine-containing herbal remedies for more than 3,000 years. Scientists have investigated berberine's traditional use in fighting infections. Berberine extracts demonstrate significant antimicrobial activity against a variety of organisms, including bacteria like Chlamydia, viruses, fungi, and protozoans.

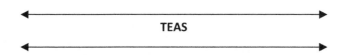

TEAS

I make up about a 3/4 gallon and store it in the refrigerator. This lasts me about 3-4 days. To simplify things, I make three teas based on the steep time. After I've made the three teas, I mix them together.

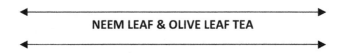

NEEM LEAF & OLIVE LEAF TEA

Ingredients
    4 cups water
    2 tsp neem leaf
    2-4 tsp olive leaf

Directions
Bring water to a boil. Add in neem leaf and olive leaf. Cover and steep for 3-4 minutes. Strain.

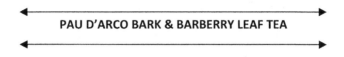
PAU D'ARCO BARK & BARBERRY LEAF TEA

Ingredients
    4 cups water
    2 tsp pau d'arco bark
    2-4 tsp barberry leaf

Directions
Bring water to a boil. Add in pau d'arco bark and barberry leaf. Cover and steep for 5-10 minutes. Strain.

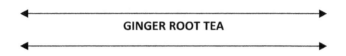
GINGER ROOT TEA

Ginger root is readily available in the vegetable section of most grocery stores. The roots are typically about 1 inch in diameter and a 2-inch section should yield about 2 tablespoons of sliced ginger.

Ingredients
    4 cups water
    4 tablespoons ginger root (fresh, raw, about 4 inches of ginger root)
    Optional: 1 tablespoon fresh lime juice (juice of 1/2 lime)

Directions
First, prepare the fresh ginger. Use a spoon and remove the skin. I used to use a peeler, but it's a lot easier to use a spoon to scrape off the skin. Cut the ginger into thin slices.

Boil the ginger in water for at least 10 minutes. For a stronger and tangier tea, allow to boil for 20 minutes or more, and use more ginger.

Remove it from the heat and add the lime juice.

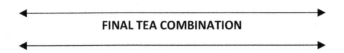

FINAL TEA COMBINATION

At this point, I mix all three teas together into 1-gallon glass jug and store in the refrigerator.

With the tea readily available, I add about 10-20 ounces of tea to my bottle of water, and I do this about three times a day.

I don't drink this tea all the time, only once in a while. It is very bitter tasting, but I feel it is beneficial.

Chapter 2

I believe the simple fact that I had begun my fight by starting to combat the disease, I mentally took on a more positive view of being able to feel better, not defeating the disease but feeling better in the process. The mind and body are so connected that I needed to form a union with body and mind if I had any chance of obtaining a better quality of life, which was my primary goal. So now every morning when I awoke I was searching to find answers on what could possibly help me, and not giving full power to the Coccidioidomycosis.

Also now I had a new mantra, 'The only *bad* action-is *no* action.'

Humans universally share some common characteristics. As humans with the disease of Valley Fever, we share common characteristics of some of the same symptoms. Basically, how we contracted this disease is 'we were in the wrong place at the wrong time', end of story! And since the doctors don't have the answers, and there is no known cure we have to look to each other who share the same problem to find a solution.

I had added fresh coconut to my hydration regimen. Hammering a nail into the coconut allowed me to get the milk, which was approximately 6 to 8 ounces. I would add the milk to my water or just drink it straight. Then I would take the hammer and shatter the hard coconut shell into smaller pieces, allowing me to use a butter knife and separate the meat from the shell. Having a container in the refrigerator of fresh coconut allowed me to chew pieces throughout the day. Coconut has a healing property of reducing cramps as well as a good source of hydration.

It was summer now, and this summer although I live in Southern California was warmer than usual. This made drinking so much water throughout the day easier. Also, I noticed my bone pain had diminished a *little* bit from the warmth. I still was not physically up to any major activity, but I would lie in the sun on my brick walkway and sweat. I immediately noticed a change in how I felt. This started to restore my enthusiasm to get better and open my mind by trying different remedies. By process of elimination, as well as trial and error, I could see myself going in a positive direction physically. I actually started visualizing myself as better. Visualization is something I always naturally had; I used it in sports growing up so I had belief in the benefits.

I visualized myself coming back to my good ol' use to be. Visualization for me, is seeing myself doing something, completing something, and in this case, feeling better before it actually happens.

Somehow, it was just a positive tool to see the result before it happened. I had become increasingly open-minded and open to new ideas in all areas of my health. Even though this was a very small 'getting better' experience, and I only saw a very small difference, I had the hope to want more. Hope, along with a positive mindset, and my visualization of getting better completed the brain part of my mind body connection. Some days it was still a struggle, but I knew if I could keep positivity at least 51% on bad days and the struggle at 49%, I was still going in the right direction to get better.

I continued taking the vitamin D twice a week, but stopped the fluconazole by personal choice. I am not a doctor, nor do I claim to be one. I'm only sharing my personal experience. And the reason I stopped the fluconazole was simple, the side effects were outweighing the benefits. Once again this is only coming from my personal experience. You will have to decide for yourself, with your doctor, what works the best for you.

So it was now time to get the body going in the same direction as my mind was, with positivity and healing. This would give me that union of mind-body that I talked about earlier. I started getting my food from the farmer's market, various forms of fruits, varieties of vegetables, fresh daily made juices and anything basically that I thought could *possibly* help me. Angie (girlfriend) would make the trip to the local farmer's market in my area. I still was having a hard time standing, or even walking small distances without extreme tiredness and general uncomfortableness. So I wasn't leaving my house much at this time. But at home I was blending foods together in my juicer in hopes of being able to feel any other way than the way I was feeling. I would mix kale with apples, watermelon, carrots and so on. Not all combinations tasted good, with some actually tasting very terrible. But I was starting to do this on a daily basis, along with roasted vegetables like cauliflower, brussels sprouts, onions and such. Since most of my life I've eaten pretty healthy it wasn't a big adaption for me to exclusively eat these foods. And my brain would tell me if you need to sacrifice flavor for health it's a very logical 'no-brainer', so just keep doing it.

When I started this new concentration of foods on a scale of 1 to 10, I was probably about a 2 on the way I was feeling overall. Then after a short period of time, probably a week or so, on a good day I would feel on the scale at about a 3. It was the smallest of small improvement, but it was an improvement and I would take anything at this point.

I started roasting vegetables, like cauliflower or brussels sprouts with garlic. In my research, I found certain foods have certain healing properties.

- Cauliflower can help with boosting the immune system and acts as an anti-inflammatory
- Brussel sprouts are good for reducing inflammation
- Garlic is great for the heart and blood system as well as a preventative to different forms of sickness
- Olive oil is an anti-inflammatory
- Asparagus is high in vitamin K and excellent for critical body detox
- Onions help body make new cells, along with sulfur property which is an anti-inflammatory agent

Also I noticed with onion it's a great way to season things in place of salt. Giving it salt like flavor, without the negative aspects of salt.

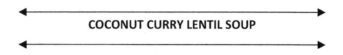

COCONUT CURRY LENTIL SOUP

Ingredients

    1 large onion
    6 garlic cloves
    1 piece ginger (approximately 3 inches)
    2 tablespoons virgin coconut oil
    5 teaspoons curry powder
    ½ teaspoon cayenne pepper
    1 can unsweetened coconut milk - 13.5-ounce
    1 cup split red lentils
    ½ cup unsweetened shredded coconut
    12 oz spinach (coarsely chopped)

Directions

Peel 1 onion and chop. Peel the garlic cloves, and chop finely. Peel ginger with a small spoon, and finely chop.

In a large pan, heat oil over medium. Add onion and cook, stirring often, just until translucent, 6–8 minutes.

Add garlic and ginger and cook, stirring often, until garlic is starting to turn golden, about 5 minutes.

Add curry powder and cayenne, stirring constantly, until spices are starting to stick to bottom of pot, about 1 minute.

Add coconut milk and stir to loosen spices, then stir in lentils, shredded coconut, and 5 cups water.

Bring to a boil over medium-high heat, then reduce heat to medium-low to keep soup at a gentle simmer. Cook, stirring occasionally, until lentils are broken down and soup is thickened, 25–30 minutes.

Add coarsely chopped spinach to pot and stir to combine. Simmer another 5 minutes.

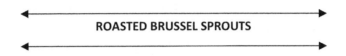

ROASTED BRUSSEL SPROUTS

Note: Exact measurements are NOT required here. I just eye ball it.

Ingredients

> 10-15 brussels sprouts, washed, ends trimmed, cut in half (or quarters if sprouts are large)
> 4 Tbsp. olive oil
> ½ teaspoon freshly ground black pepper
> 3-4 grated garlic cloves (more if you want)
> Red red pepper flakes (optional)
> Pine nuts (optional)

Directions

Preheat oven to 400° F. Line a baking sheet with parchment paper.

In a medium bowl, combine olive oil, black pepper, red pepper flakes and grated garlic. I like using a ceramic garlic grater. Mix together. Add brussel sprouts and toss until all sprouts are coated with olive oil mixture. (If you want to avoid washing more dishes, place everything in a large re-sealable plastic bag. Seal tightly, and shake to coat.)

Pour onto prepared baking sheet, and place on center oven rack.

Roast for 15 minutes, turn each brussel sprout over and cook for another 15 minutes. During the last 15 minutes of cooking, I make the sauce.

Cook until tender. They should be browed and caramelized on the bottom and edges. If they look like they are burning, reduce the oven temperature to 350 degrees.

Top with Spicy Aioli Sauce (recipe below) and pine nuts. Serve immediately.

ROASTED CAULIFLOWER STEAKS

Ingredients

> 1 large head cauliflower, sliced lengthwise through the core into 4 'steaks'
> ¼ cup olive oil
> 1 tablespoon fresh lemon juice
> 2-4 cloves garlic, minced or grated
> 1 pinch red pepper flakes, or to taste
> Ground black pepper to taste

Directions

Preheat oven to 400° F. Line a baking sheet with parchment paper.

Place cauliflower steaks on the prepared baking sheet.

Whisk olive oil, lemon juice, garlic, red pepper flakes, and black pepper together in a bowl. Brush half of the olive oil mixture over the tops of the cauliflower steaks.

Roast cauliflower steaks in the preheated oven for 15 minutes. Gently turn over each steak and brush with remaining olive oil mixture. Continue roasting until tender and golden, 15 to 20 minutes more.

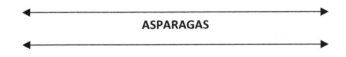

ASPARAGAS

Ingredients

    1 pound medium asparagus
    1 to 2 tablespoons extra-virgin olive oil
    Freshly ground pepper
    1 lemon, cut into wedges

Directions

To prepare asparagus, snap the cut end off each stalk. The asparagus automatically breaks just where the woody part ends and the fresh, juicy asparagus begins. So you don't need to worry about breaking off too much or too little.

Pour about 1-inch of water into a large saucepan, and set up a collapsible steamer inside. If you don't have a steamer, use less water and simply place the spears directly in the water. Bring the water to boil, lay the asparagus in the steamer, cover, and steam until crisp-tender, about 4 to 5 minutes. If the spears are small, reduce the steam time to 2-3 minutes. Asparagus is better under cooked than over cooked. Remove from pan and drizzle with olive oil or melted butter (I use unsalted. I personally feel salt is our enemy.)

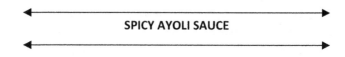

SPICY AYOLI SAUCE

Ingredients

    ½ c. mayonnaise
    Juice of half lemon
    ½ tsp. cayenne pepper

In a small bowl mix together mayonnaise, lemon juice, and cayenne pepper.

Pour on top of roasted vegetables.

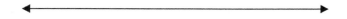

    Roasted vegetables and lentils are a staple in our household. To avoid the monotony of flavor, I use many different sauces and seasonings. I keep the healing properties of the spices at the forefront of my mind to make sure I am feeding my health, not the disease.

Chapter 3

It gets very tedious washing and cutting vegetables, and I started to find easier ways of doing things. For example, I started buying the Christopher Ranch brand of already peeled and lightly roasted garlic. It comes in a 6 ounce package, with approximately 7 individually wrapped pods of roasted garlic weighing 170 g each. Each pod is good for one or two meals. With garlic's healing properties of benefiting heart and blood filtering, I started to make this the cornerstone of most of my meals.

Snacking on nuts throughout the day is something I've always done, and after researching nuts (any type) I found that nuts are extremely good for health in general, good for brain function as well as helping with depression. And I personally believe that a certain amount of depression comes from being in pain every day caused from this Valley Fever. Naturally I buy the unsalted and in bulk, which most major supermarkets carry now. Also almond butter, peanut butter, cashew butter has the same benefits as eating raw nuts when you purchase these butter products at supermarkets that carry the 'grind your own kind'. It's simply a machine with raw nuts and you place a container under it, push a button and you have a spreadable form of nuts with no salt, no sugar and less than half the price of brand name. Most wholesale supermarkets have these options so it's well worth finding one that offers this form of nut-butter.

I knew I needed to find something physically to do to get me moving around in some form. At this point walking, running or any type of calisthenics was not feasible, so I came up with swimming. My buddy Lester owns a condo with a pool and gave me an access key so I could swim anytime I wanted. Since your body weighs less in water, common sense told me it would be easier to move around and receive the benefits of good exercise with the least resistance. At first, believe me I was doing more floating than swimming, but with time I would slowly take a lap or two. Staying consistent I would find myself able to do more and more. I wasn't going to break any swimming records because I still would get winded and extremely tired, but I was doing something and this I put on my list of positive to-dos. And on that pain scale of 1 to 10, I was at a solid 4 on most days, and just as negativity breeds negativity, positivity started breeding positivity.

My mind and body were in sync. When eating well my brain would remind me to swim, after swimming my body would remind my brain to eat well. After a warm day in the pool, I would make a salad out of kale, spinach, avocados and sliced jalapeno. I would use olive oil for the salad dressing, and maybe some crumbled cheese for flavor. Adding some sunflower seeds, which are in the nut family, I would make a satisfying lunch.

- Kale is an extremely nutritionally dense food group and contains antioxidants as well

- Spinach is considered a *Superfood,* with one of the major benefits of being good for *respiratory* health.
- Avocados maintain electrical gradients (balance) in body cells and excellent for kidney function
- Jalapenos help with arthritis and *pain relief* (not all jalapenos are spicy hot. You can get the 'tamed' version and they have the same benefits)

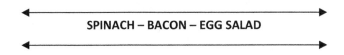

SPINACH – BACON – EGG SALAD

Ingredients

2 cloves garlic
½ teaspoon sea salt
2 tablespoons red wine vinegar
1 tablespoon Dijon
3 Tablespoons extra-virgin olive oil
Freshly ground pepper to taste
12 cups spinach leaves
4 eggs, hard boiled (see tips below*) peeled and chopped
4 slices bacon, cooked crispy, cooled and crumbled

Instructions

Dressing: Peel garlic cloves. Grate with ceramic garlic grater. Mix with salt to form a paste. Scrape into a medium bowl. Whisk in vinegar and Dijon. Gradually whisk in oil. Season with pepper.

Place spinach, eggs and bacon in a large salad bowl. Pour dressing over the salad and toss to combine.

Hard-Boiled Egg Instructions

Place your raw eggs in a medium saucepan and cover with at least 2 inches of cold water. You need to fully cover eggs with at least 2 inches of water for this to work. Less water means that it will cool down quicker and your eggs won't cook thoroughly.

Place the pan over high heat until it reaches a boil.

Turn off heat, cover and let it sit for 13 minutes.

After 13 minutes, remove the eggs from the pan and place them in an ice-water bath and let them cool for five minutes.

Use in a recipe or store in your refrigerator.

*Hard Boiled Egg Tips

For easy to peel eggs, I suggest following these tricks:

- Fresh eggs don't peel well, so use eggs that have been in your refrigerator about a week
- After cooking, let the eggs rest in an ice-bath to "shock" them.
- Refrigerated hard-boiled eggs will not peel well. Peel your eggs once they have cooled down to room temperature.

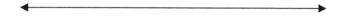

Over my lifetime, I've seen a lot of changes in food, from the processing to the taste being different from how certain foods tasted when I was young. My biggest observation would be meats tasting noticeably different than I remember as a kid. I stopped eating steak as well as hamburger many years ago from personal choice for no other reason than the lack of flavor. But I would crave Italian sausage as well as salami, and enjoyed a sliced turkey sandwich once in a while. I started observing that any form of lunchmeat, even the most expensive brand, would take away from my well-being. And the richness of sausages and processed salami wouldn't agree with me either. After a little time passing with my eating so clean and calculated, certain outside foods would immediately cause a reaction. Hard to put my finger on exactly how it made me feel, the only way I can best describe it is that it seem to be taking away from the direction of me feeling better. This is just a personal observation that I wanted to add in case someone else experiences the same situation.

A lot of life for me is trial and error along with observing what happens when I do this, what doesn't happen when I don't do that. It's no more than figuring out a personal way, or plan, of doing something.

I believe most humans are all on a path to achieve a better quality-of-life. What we choose and don't choose for our way of doing things makes our path personal, but we all have a universal destination. For myself, I eliminated most meats from my diet long before my Valley Fever diagnosis. I would still eat grilled chicken, salmon, or tuna, and once in a while I like to have some sausage or salami, but usually eat this at home because I prefer a lower sodium, higher quality product.

I love the art of breaking bread with friends. Some of the best times I have are having meals out while laughing and talking about life with my close-knit friends. Just the overall sitting down, sharing a meal and exchanging views is a satisfying part of my life. But I had to change drastically where I would eat and what I would eat while dining out. I'm a big fan of Mexican food and found a restaurant that I really enjoy dining at for many years now. I would order the same thing every time, a bean and cheese burrito with onions, cilantro and grilled jalapenos. The salsa and chips are homemade, making this one of my favorite places to eat. After this extremely delicious Mexican dish, I would get that feeling of something not being exactly right again, noticeably causing my Valley Fever symptoms to flare up. But I noticed even though the chips are homemade I wouldn't feel exactly right after eating them; I surmised this must be the oil they use to cook the chips in. So naturally I stopped eating the chips and the negative physical feeling went away.

My keen awareness of how much my bones would ache, headaches, muscle cramps and nose running would fluctuate based on the foods. This let me know that I was on to something. I fine-tuned my process of food addition as well as food elimination to more narrow down how I felt on a daily basis. Literally I could keep track of the degree of pain immediately after I ate something that didn't fit into my new food regimen, and if it didn't increase my symptoms right away, the next morning I would know for sure that it was not something I should have eaten. This gave me the hope to go on investigating what I needed to do to feel even better. I was noticing big improvements in my pain levels but it wasn't enough. I knew doing little things created little relief, doing more would create more relief. This is the first time that my hope for a better quality-of-life was now a definite attainable goal.

On my *initial* visit before my Valley Fever diagnosis my general practitioner had noticed a hernia in my groin area, which he said I would need surgery for. He referred me to a local surgeon after my cocci diagnosis that specialized in hernia repairs. After my initial consultation appointment with the surgeon, the surgery doctor who was going to perform this minor operation informed me that I wasn't healthy enough to be operated on because of the state I was in due to the Coccidioidomycosis. My oxygen levels, recent blood tests and x-rays put me at risk, so the doctor did not want me to undergo the hernia repair surgery.

After this short time window of change, only about maybe three months, of attacking the Valley Fever in the manner of changes that I was making with light exercise and food choices, the surgeon cleared me to have this procedure done. He also said he was somewhat taken aback by my speedy progress, especially since I was off the fluconazole. This felt like a milestone in the sense that getting better was becoming more of a reality instead of *maybe* something I'd only conjured up with my positive mindset. Knowing the evidence of my current tests showed improvement, this reinforcement created more focus to find ways of even greater improvement.

There was still some summer-like days left and with the warm weather I was now enjoying more of life in general, with the swimming and reduced pain. I decided to not schedule my hernia repair surgery until the late fall of the year. Knowing I would be laid up for a number of weeks physically, healing from my operation, and wanted to enjoy more of my newfound feeling. Make no mistake I was still in pain but this is where the mind part of that partnership, mind-body, lifted my body up for that little boost I needed to continue the physical portion of that partnership, that I believe is crucial in positive results.

Although the surgery went without a hitch the recovery process was brutal. The first two weeks any form of movement was severely painful, and even though the doctor told me six weeks for full recovery, my anesthesiologist, who had had a similar operation informed me that it was probably closer to twelve weeks for the full recovery process. But during this time is when I gained the most knowledge on the do's and don'ts of Valley Fever.

The first weeks of the healing process from my hernia surgery overshadowed the pain my body was feeling from the Valley Fever. Then I realized how I had been cutting corners with my eating, mostly out of convenience and a little laziness. I don't have a natural sweet tooth, but during these times it was the holidays. I would find myself eating a couple of homemade cookies, or a slice of pie with ice cream. This was not the usual for me, but the next morning after my *sweet tooth* indulging, I would pay the price. Getting out of bed in the mornings was extremely painful again, and it'd been months since that type of pain attacked my bones. So I said no more sugar... in any form.

I've known people during my entire life that are completely healthy, and after quitting sugar they would feel better. So if no sugar for a healthy person helps, no sugar for a sick person would help also. Although sugar has never been my weakness, I started putting all foods that I ate under my microscope of thinking to eliminate from my diet completely if they contained sugar. I started subtracting fresh fruit first, although they contain *natural* sugar when all is said and done the body interprets the fruit as sugar. Out went apples, tangerines, blueberries and others, even the dried fruit. Dried cranberries, dried apricots that I had been putting into my mixed nuts for flavor had to go also. Watermelon had become one of my main sources of fruit to turn into a juice, and I even eliminated that.

Now I would only use the rind portion of the watermelon, mixed with ice to make a refreshing smoothie. Watermelon rinds open up the blood vessels, making easier blood flow as well as another form of boosting the immune system all without sugar.

Most people throw out watermelon rind and eat only the red portion, but watermelon rind contains more of the amino acid citrulline than the pink flesh. Not only do watermelon rinds contain all the same nutrients as is found in the juicy fruit, but even higher concentrations of certain antioxidants, minerals, vitamins, and active ingredients. This tough rind contains low levels of calories, but high concentrations of vitamin C, vitamin A, vitamin B6, potassium, and zinc, among others. Watermelon rind is also nutrient dense with chlorophyll, citrulline, lycopene, amino acids, and flavonoids and phenolic compounds.

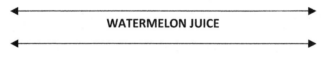

WATERMELON JUICE

Ingredients

> Watermelon rinds
> A thumb-size piece of ginger (optional)

A little piece of ginger makes this juice a little spicy. You can skip the ginger if you wish. This herb root is excellent for stomach health.

Wash your watermelon and lemon before cutting.

Use a spoon to remove the skin from the ginger.

Cut off the watermelon rind and chop into pieces that will fit the mouth of your juicer. Run them through. Cut the lemon into quarters. Run it through. Chop ginger into several pieces and run through.

Stir everything together. Store in refrigerator.

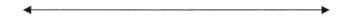

I even subtracted from my eating some of the vegetables that I felt contained too much sugar causing the vegetable portion of benefits to be outweighed by the sugar content, foods like beets, carrots, even tomatoes.

My laziness came in the form of not having readily available (quality food) on hand at those times that I became hungry. All these recipes and ideas are great, but when you get hungry you want something quick, easy and accessible. I'm human and when I get hungry I will grab the first thing available to eat, even if it's something that I don't feel is the best choice at that time. So what I would do is find more convenient ways of preparation of certain foods, and or mixing up something in the morning that I could eat throughout the day. The farmer's market would only be on Saturday morning, and sometimes it wasn't convenient to shop then. I started investigating the supermarkets and realized they offer a lot of good foods in a more convenient manner. I would buy bags of shredded broccoli, fresh washed spinach for easy preparation and availability.

One of my favorite food mixes that I keep on hand most of the time is a combination of tuna, roasted garlic, pickled jalapenos with shredded broccoli. I would also add some of my mixed nut combo for flavor and texture. I was even buying *slivered* almonds instead of whole almonds to mix with the sunflower seeds, *quartered* walnuts and pecans to make the mix more subtle when added to other combinations of food.

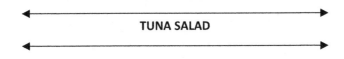

TUNA SALAD

Ingredients

    1 can of albacore tuna in water (12 oz can)
    2 medium avocados
    ¼ cup pickled jalapenos (to taste/optional)
    1 pod roasted garlic
    ½ cup shredded broccoli
    ¼ cup mixed nuts

Drain the can of albacore tuna. Peel and remove avocado seed. Mix all ingredients together in a bowl. Refrigerate.

Throughout the day I can grab a couple of spoonfuls of the tuna mix, so I don't get off course because of my hunger.

Also I may put in some hummus for flavor. Personally, I use hummus in a lot of my vegetable mixes to pull it all together. It is nothing more than chickpeas with a little seasoning and comes in a variety of flavors. It's really a nice way of bringing taste variety to familiar dishes.

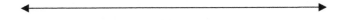

Chapter 4

After recouping from my surgery, I needed to get physical again. With the kicking involved in swimming, along with public pool water, I didn't feel this would be good at the time with having a fresh incision, plus I would have to travel 3 miles to go to my friends' pool. The doctor told me to walk as far as I felt comfortable, so I would walk a block or so at first. But I lacked purpose at this time and needed to find something that would motivate me to move around more. So I decided to get a puppy, an American Staffordshire who weighed 4 pounds. This is an active breed of dog and when fully grown would weigh about 65 pounds.

I named him Joe (like I name all my dogs since I was a child) and Joe became my purpose. There's an old saying about having a dog, 'it will keep you young.' I realize not everyone is an animal person and/or their lifestyle won't allow them to have a pet. My point is to find the *purpose* to get up and move around within your own life, that does not require the actual mental push from yourself, but a *purpose* that requires your physical involvement. I realized that every day I would have to spend time walking with Joe along with his rapid growth and need for more activity. This would cause me to have more activity in my own life. Simple; my personal *purpose*!

Finding your *personal* purpose is key, not only for the physical aspect but this is also a great positive motivator to get yourself doing more. With my mind open to new ideas I went out of my comfort zone by doing hot yoga, 104° with 40% humidity. Believe me this was out of my comfort zone but the benefits were amazing. Not so much the yoga poses themselves since I wasn't very yoga savvy, but the purpose of having to be involved to the best of my abilities, which would still cause me to sweat profusely. Sitting in a sauna is another good way to achieve success in getting rid of the poisons within our bodies. This became another discovery of mine, that sweating a little or a lot in any way shape or form is beneficial to how I feel.

Consistency and moderation was a nice starting point for me. My dog was young and didn't need much walking at first but I knew with his growth and active breed that during his growing, I would be taking on more walking and activity at the same pace.

With my newfound *purpose* I became optimistic and hopeful even more so. Purpose is everything. This is when I first realized in my heart of hearts that if I would put all the components together I could achieve major strides in my quality of life. Not letting the Valley Fever own my life nor control my mind, I was taking all the power away from the disease and channeling everything towards a solution. I believe it was Socrates who said, "There is no such thing as wisdom… only *repetition*."

So every morning when I would wake up, I started to repeat the same actions. This gave me a positive routine which became my foundation for that quality of life I was striving for.

My aloe water mix first thing, then I would take time to *visualize* walking further than I had the day before, and I had my *purpose*, Joe the dog, to motivate me to start moving. Also I started doing the food shopping for me and Angie, I would notice that certain foods that I was used to and crave started to look more as pain, then as satisfying. Angie didn't eat exactly like I did, so I would buy her favorite foods for her also.

For me food ended up into two categories. First there was the food that I felt was causing me problems, and second, the healing food. It was real simple. I had become tired of eating all this healthy healing food that I had discovered only to crave a pint of ice cream at night or some other snack food I felt like I couldn't live without, then giving in to my craving. I was taking two steps forward and one step back with the trade-off defining how I felt. So now I looked at healing foods exclusively to eat, I even stopped eating breads, pasta, oatmeal and rice, also no crackers or any other foods that would cause me to feel full before I got to the healing food that I felt my body truly needed. Now I'm a guy that likes pasta and a good heated French bread with butter, but I knew I had to stop so I could load my body with more of the healing foods that I discovered for pain relief.

After a couple weeks, I wasn't really missing the foods that I was accustomed to and immediately started to feel better. My energy increased also and I depended on olive oil, avocados and nuts along with nut butter for my energy source. My walks with Joe were limited at first to about a block or two, but my constant visualization of walking more was pushing me in that positive manner that I needed to focus on. Where I live there are some hills above my house. This area is developed with homes and streets, and the degree of slopes and steepness vary. I would visualize myself walking these hills and was determined to push myself into this new challenge.

I've been taking 800 mg of ibuprofen every morning and late in the afternoon for many years. The aches and pains in my joints I had attributed to being so athletic during my entire life and now that I was sixty-seven years old I felt the aches and pains went with the territory of age. But I made one of my goals to cut down on the ibuprofen intake, or even cut out completely ibuprofen. This felt impossible but I was very driven at this point, I felt like I was on to something that was definitely going to be a game changer in how I felt on a daily basis. So I kept eating and walking with only one thing on my mind and that was to get better, and I noticed that I was. I was experiencing very small signs of improvement, but it was improvement all the same and I definitely wanted more.

The other changes that did occur were the spotty rash that was on my legs and torso had completely disappeared, and my nose was running a lot less. I have learned that the biggest indicator on how I'm doing is the volume of how much my nose runs. The first time I walked a half mile, at my own pace, I felt as if I had conquered the Appalachian Trail. The hills above my house were my next project. Also I stopped juicing almost completely since the solid foods seem to be a better choice. Lightly cooked and in their rawest form created the best results. Finding new recipes made better choices for a variety of good foods without the ho-hum repetitive menu. One of my favorites became cauliflower crust pizza.

CAULIFLOWER PIZZA CRUST

This makes one pizza, so I double the recipe to make two.

A cauliflower pizza crust will not rise since there is no yeast involved, and since the crust is entirely cauliflower, cheese, and egg, it will not achieve the same crispness as a thin dough pizza. But the pizza will stay together just fine, and will taste very much like a pizza.

Ingredients

> 1 medium head of cauliflower (6" – 7" wide or 2.5–3 lbs.)
> 1 egg beaten
> 1 tsp Italian seasoning (dried oregano or basil)
> ¼ tsp ground black pepper
> 1 cup of freshly grated Parmesan cheese
> ½ cup Mozzarella cheese, grated/shredded
> Optional: 1/8 tsp salt. We don't usually add any salt
>
> PIZZA TOPPINGS
> Your choice. We like basil, mozzarella, peppers and spinach.

Preheat oven to 400° F. Line a baking sheet with parchment paper.

Grate fresh cauliflower florets.

Heat the grated cauliflower in a skillet—don't add oil or water—use medium heat, not too hot. Stir regularly. Cook until the cauliflower has dried out somewhat, about 10 minutes. Remove skillet from heat and set aside to allow cauliflower to cool slightly.

In a bowl, beat 1 egg. Add Italian seasoning and grated Parmesan cheese. You can substitute, with any other hard cheese like asiago or Romano.

Add the cauliflower to the bowl and mix well with the egg and cheese and form into a ball.

Place the balled cauliflower and cheese onto the parchment paper and spread out into a pizza shape about ¼ inch thick. The crust will be about 10" across.

Do not make the edges of the crust too thin; keep the size of the crust uniform for even cooking. The cauliflower will darken quite rapidly around the edges if too thin.

Place crust into an oven preheated to 400 degrees and cook approx. 15-20 minutes until the crust has browned and firmed up.

Remove cauliflower pizza crust from the oven and top with your favorite pizza sauce. Use a pesto, white sauce, or whatever. We don't always use sauce, and it is delicious either way. Top with your favorite pizza toppings.

Return pizza to the oven and continue to cook at 400 F for about 10 minutes until the toppings are done, watch the edges of the cauliflower crust; the edges will darken too much if overcooked.

Treat it like a pizza. Slice and enjoy.

GARLIC PARMESAN SPAGHETTI SQUASH

Ingredients

    8 tablespoons unsalted butter, divided
    3 cloves garlic, minced
    ¼ cup low-sodium vegetable broth
    ½ cup freshly grated Parmesan
    2 tablespoons chopped fresh parsley leaves

FOR THE SPAGHETTI SQUASH
    1 (2-3 pounds) spaghetti squash
    2 tablespoons olive oil
    Sea salt and freshly ground black pepper, to taste

Directions

Preheat oven to 375° F. Line a baking sheet with parchment paper.

You will need a well-sharpened knife. Cut the squash in half lengthwise from stem to tail and scrape out the seeds. Drizzle with olive oil and season with salt and pepper, to taste.

Place squash, cut-side down, onto the prepared baking sheet. Place into oven and roast until tender, about 35-45 minutes.

Remove from oven and let rest until cool enough to handle.

Using a fork, scrape the flesh to create long strands.

Melt 4 tablespoons butter in a large skillet over medium high heat. Add garlic, and cook, stirring frequently, until fragrant, about 1 minute.

Stir in vegetable broth. Bring to a boil; reduce heat and simmer until reduced by half, about 1-2 minutes. Stir in remaining 4 tablespoons butter, 1 tablespoon at a time, until melted and smooth.

Stir in spaghetti squash and gently toss to combine until heated through, about 2 minutes.

Serve immediately, topped with Parmesan and garnished with parsley, if desired.

Chapter 5

My progress now turned into success but success did not come overnight. The changes that I was experiencing kept me motivated and on track. When Joe the dog would give me that look and remind me of my *purpose*, which was to walk farther and more I would get up and go. Everything was starting to click at this point and I started looking forward to being a little better than the previous day. Staying open-minded, I signed up for a course that my good friend Steve Dillon offered. He founded a program which offers brain revitalization and he lectures in seminars across the country.

His brain course teaches us to eliminate the loop that we have in our thinking, this loop is a negative thought coming after a positive idea or start. This *habitual* loop, as Steve says causes us not to venture out and succeed at most things we attempt by fear stemming from doubt from previous experience, this puts our brain in default mode. He teaches this program to enabling families, people with addiction disorders, corporate executives, and many others. So I felt this could be something I need also to make that union of mind-body stronger. So I took his "Vision and Future Focus" program. The primary purpose of the course is to *connect people with purpose and potential*. This tremendously helped me and made me fully realize failing was not an option and remaining sick was unacceptable. I not only could, but I would conquer my Coccidioidomycosis. Please don't misunderstand me I'm not saying that I could cure the Valley Fever, but I could arrest the symptoms and continue on my one true path, a quality-of-life.

For more information: www.sdillonconsulting.com

My walks became my daily physical commitment and within a short period of time, I was trekking up to 2 miles per walk. Although it was taxing my body I noticed that my joint pain was subsiding, muscle cramps were completely gone. I was experiencing tiredness, not so much from the disease but from the exercise. I actually started feeling really well when I would push myself. The hills above my house became part of my physical routine, and although the hills were very challenging, I could walk them once in a while at my own pace. On a good day I would naturally speed up my walking, on a not so good day I would take it slow. Then there were days that I would be overwhelmed with the thought of walking, so I wouldn't walk. But those days became fewer and fewer. I would take Joe to the beach and let him chase his tennis ball endlessly, and since I was the one throwing the ball this would help me benefit from even more movement.

The pain in my joints and throughout my body was dramatically disappearing. I cannot tell you what a relief this became. I even started to run short distances during my walks, and a 4-mile walk on flat ground and hills became very doable, once in a while. I was pushing, sweating and mentally driving myself to do more and it was paying off in such an indescribable manner. I had come so far from that guy that was sitting on the couch crippled in pain overcome with mental anguish with no direction and the constant thought of coming to the end of life's road. To help you with the insight of the despair that I felt at first, I had taken the time to say a heartfelt goodbye to Angie with a life reflecting perspective on her deep importance of love and friendship to me in my life. Dark times for sure. But now the comparison was night and day. This was definitely a fight to get where I am today, at sixty-eight years old, to how I was when diagnosed with Valley Fever at sixty five. But when I look back in hindsight I feel that the complacency of my physical being during the dark times could not have been helped, but now I have no excuse since I found a combination of relatively small things that I can do on a daily basis that would and will make me better.

I even added more to my exercise routine with light dumbbells for an upper body workout, stretching, and also found another *tool* to help me. I bought a yoga tube which is 36 inches long, 6 inches in diameter made out of polyurethane. The brand I bought is YES 4 ALL but I'm sure other companies make them also. And what I do is lay lengthways with my spine centered on the tube and let gravity spread my rib cage by pulling my shoulders down. I recommend this inexpensive helpful tool to everyone strongly. I also turn it sideways and roll back and forth from my tailbone to my neck. These exercises align your spine and make walking and other movement noticeably easier. With increased exercise I felt my body needed more carbohydrates than the ones that I was only getting with vegetables so I came up with a mix that not only is easy to prepare and comes in handy to have in the refrigerator to snack on whenever.

I keep lentils in the refrigerator and add shredded broccoli, mixed nuts, hummus, roasted garlic, or whatever my taste at the moment craves. I eat them cold or hot. They have a neutral taste, so their flavor doesn't override any other foods you may add with them.

I have experimented with different lentils and found that the green and brown lentils hold together best when cooked. Yellow, red, and orange lentils taste good, but since they tend to get mushy when cooked, they are better for soups and sauces rather than cooked on their own.

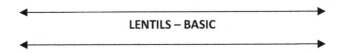

LENTILS – BASIC

Be sure to use a large enough saucepan as the lentils will double or triple in size.

I used to cook them with a low-sodium vegetable broth, but I found out that this was making them tough. I would overcook them in hopes they would become tender, but they would go from tough to mush.

I learned that cooking with stock or broth made the lentils crunchy even when fully cooked. So instead of cooking with stock, I use plain water and add the salt when they are done cooking. If you stir in the salt while the lentils are still warm, they will absorb just enough to taste fully seasoned. Personally, I use sea salt.

Every recipe I found calls for rinsing the uncooked lentils in a colander or strain before cooking, but honestly I have never done this.

Ingredients

1 large onion
2 tablespoons olive oil
3 cups of water
1 cup dry lentils (green or brown)
Pinch of salt

Directions

Peel onion and chop. In a large pan, heat oil over medium. Add onion and cook, stirring often. Cook until onions are translucent, about 6–8 minutes.

Add 3 cups of water and 1 cup of dry lentils. Bring to a boil, reduce heat and simmer and cover. Cook about 25-30 minutes, or until they are tender. Remove from heat, add a pinch of salt and stir. Cover and let set for a couple of minutes to let salt absorb.

This is where you can be creative and make dishes of your own. For a taste change, instead of lentils, I use beans. My go-to's are black beans (low sodium) and vegetarian refried beans. Whenever I use canned beans, I pour the beans into a colander and rinse before I use them.

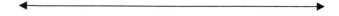

Noticing my muscle tone improving and the loss of 15 pounds in my body weight, from exercise and my eating ritual, and these are definitely pounds that needed shedding. I started feeling unstoppable at this point. I had no stress or worry on my physical being, and as I've always said, 'Stress and worry is nothing more than meditation on negativity.' I cut my morning Advil in half (200 milligrams) and very rarely took any in the afternoon or early evening. Some mornings I would forget to take the 200 mg of Advil and wouldn't even notice. Big changes for sure.

Although I'm not a big red meat guy out of choice, I know a lot of people are, so here's an easy recipe that's tasty. This is the only red meat I eat for no other reason than it reminds me of how steak used to taste as a kid.

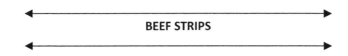

BEEF STRIPS

Ingredients

Taco seasoning
½ cup Liquid aminos
1 lb. flap meat, approximately three-quarter inch thick

Directions

If you have time, you can marinate overnight, but it isn't necessary.

Preheat oven to 250° or lower. Slow cooking is the secret for tender and tasty meat.

Cut meat into 1" strips. Mix taco seasoning and liquid amino in a zip lock bag. Add meat to bag and coat with seasoning. Place meat on a pan and into the oven. Cook slowly, flipping meat once in a while. Cook to your preference of doneness.

Or you can barbeque them which is a great way to bring out the flavor. Again, low temperature and slow cooking is key.

Refrigerate.

CONCLUSION

The sole reason for writing this book was to *show others change is possible*.

I've drawn from personal experience and personal success to write this book. I kept it simple and condensed because it is important to understand what caused my changes. I started out with blind faith which became hope. My positivity allowed me to realize that life is to be enjoyed which opened my mind to new ideas so I can obtain a better quality-of-life regardless of my Valley Fever. My positive mental attitude no longer allows me to accept sitting on the couch, looking out my window and watching the world pass me by.

I spoke earlier that as humans, we have the same universal characteristics, and we have the same personal ability to change. I know from my lowest point when the Coccidioidomycosis had me in that very dark place that I had to do something different, and I had to look outside myself. I needed to be open minded. I needed an extremely positive attitude. It is my experience that because of making relatively small changes, I experience profound change. I implore you to realize that if I can do it—you can also.

Just a few days ago I went back to my doctor for a follow-up visit, and my vitals tell the whole story of my personal change. My blood pressure was 118/82, pulse 64 beats per minute, and this is the big one, my oxygen level was 97%. At my Valley Fever starting point my oxygen was 91%, and know that oxygen levels in and around 90% are considered to be very compromised. On that scale of 1 to 10 that I talked about earlier on how I felt, I now stay at a solid 8! That is from morning to night and on a daily basis, and trust and believe when I tell you how much my life has changed. I spend time at the beach, I go camping and I don't plan my day around my disease. Doing the desires of my heart whenever I want, how ever I want, has become very liberating and enjoyable to say the least. Today I feel better compared to even years before I was diagnosed with cocci.

My hope for you is that you may take some or all of this information that I've written from personal testimony and experience, incorporate into your life, and see what happens.

Thoughts matter…If you keep reminding yourself of your limitations, they remain yours.

Appendix

BARBERRY ROOT

The Chinese have used berberine-containing herbal remedies for more than 3,000 years. Scientists have investigated berberine's traditional use in fighting infections. Berberine extracts demonstrate significant antimicrobial activity against a variety of organisms, including bacteria like Chlamydia, viruses, fungi, and protozoans.

Those who are suffering from hyperthyroid disorder and pregnant or nursing women should avoid Barberry Root extracts in any form, additionally; those who are considering taking it should be aware that some side effects include depression and lethargy as well as skin and eye irritation.

Warning: Not to be used during pregnancy. Not to be used while nursing.

NEEM LEAF

The use of neem leaves has been studied, and in 2005 scientists published a research report, Medicinal properties of neem leaves: a review. It is a compilation of existing scientific studies and clinical trials. It shows very impressively just how versatile the leaves are. Here is what it says about the benefits of neem leaves: "Neem leaf and its constituents have been demonstrated to exhibit immunomodulatory, anti-inflammatory, antihyperglycaemic, antiulcer, antimalarial, antifungal, antibacterial, antiviral, antioxidant, antimutagenic and anticarcinogenic properties."

Take neem leaf in moderation, and start with a little when trying it for the first time.

- Don't take any neem products internally if you are trying to conceive a child (this applies to women and men!) or pregnant

- Don't attempt to treat fever in children with neem

Let me repeat the last point: never give neem in any form to children with fever or viral illnesses. Neem contains Aspirin like substances, and like Aspirin, it can lead to Reye syndrome.

NOTE: Neem leaf is not the same as leaf extract. Additionally, neem oil is neem seed oil, not neem leaf oil as some people wrongly assume. It can be made safe for consumption, but neem oil really needs special knowledge and treatment before can be taken internally.

OLIVE LEAVES

Research shows oleuropein, the main component in olive leaf extract, has antioxidant, antibacterial, antimicrobial, anti-inflammatory, and immune-stimulating properties.

Olive leaf extract may interact with certain medicines. Do not take olive leaf if you are taking blood pressure medications as it may cause low blood pressure. People who are taking insulin or other blood sugar medicine also should not take olive leaf as it may cause hypoglycemia.

People who are undergoing chemotherapy should talk to their doctor before taking olive leaf extract as it may interfere with the actions of certain chemotherapy drugs due to its antioxidant properties.

PAU D' ARCO BARK

In herbal medicine, extracts of the pau d'arco bark have long been used to treat a wide range of medical disorders. The information I found pointed to it helping reduce inflammation and infection. What interested me is that the bark is highly resistant to rotting, mold, and other common tree pathogens. It has long been presumed that these antimicrobial properties may be beneficial to humans, either by preventing or treating common bacterial, viral, or fungal infections.

As with all herbal products, be careful. I read that when taken in doses larger than 1.5 grams (1,500 milligrams), pau d'arco can become toxic and cause damage to the kidneys or liver. Overuse of pau d'arco can lead to severe vomiting, abdominal pain, fainting, and bloody stools.

Pau d'arco may slow blood clotting and increase the risk of bleeding during and after surgery. Stop using pau d'arco for at least two weeks before undergoing any type of surgical procedure.

Because pau d'arco can slow blood clotting, it should not be used with anticoagulants like Coumadin (warfarin) or antiplatelet drugs like Plavix (clopidogrel).

Due to the lack of safety research, pau d'arco should not be used in children, pregnant women, or nursing mothers. It should also be used with caution in people with kidney or liver disease.

Made in the USA
Las Vegas, NV
06 March 2022